BODY SMART 101

BY LOREN SHINAULT

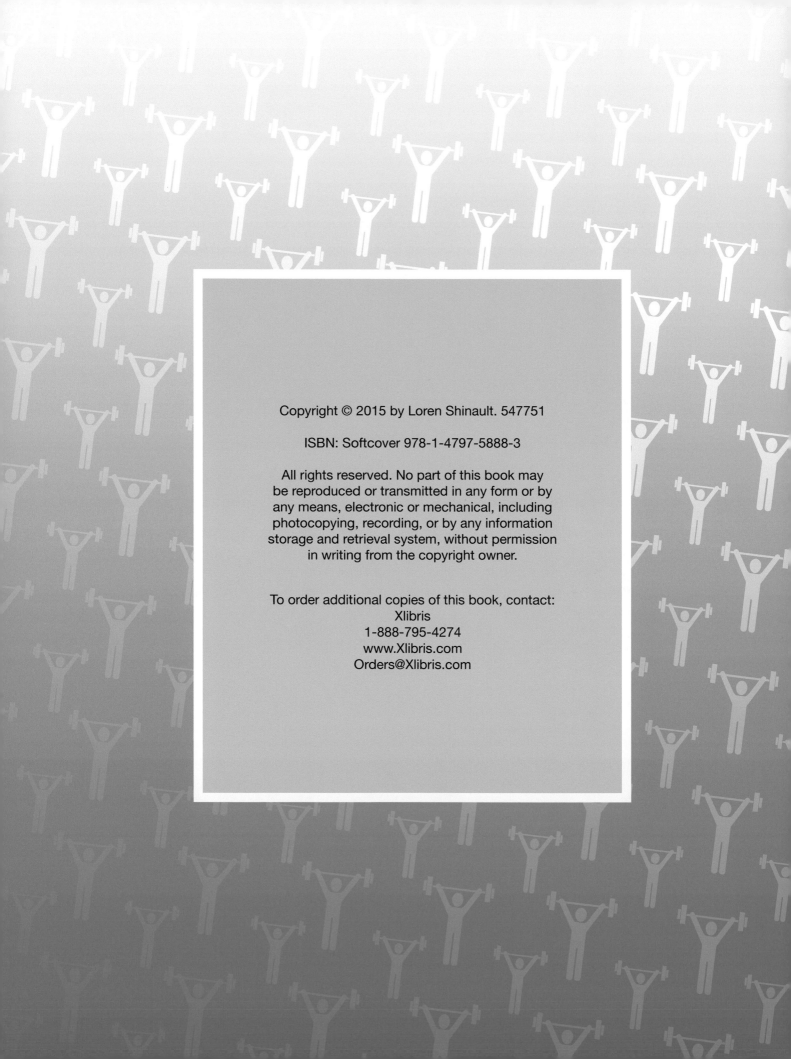

To order additional copies of this book, contact:
Xlibris
1-888-795-4274
www.Xlibris.com
Orders@Xlibris.com

BODY SMART 101

BY LOREN SHINAULT

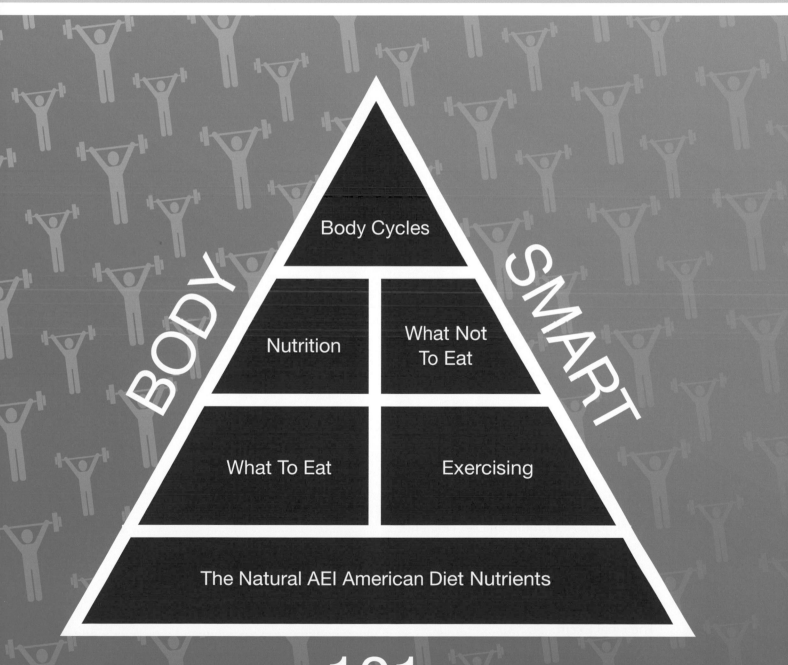

BODY

SMART

Body Cycles

Nutrition

What Not To Eat

What To Eat

Exercising

The Natural AEI American Diet Nutrients

101

INDEX

CHAPTER 1
BODY CYCLES

Body Smart was written to do just that, make your body smart. By you learning a few things about your body and changing several bad habits into good ones you will be much healthier.

Body cycles are the first things we need to discuss. Our bodies go through three cycles a day.

1. Elimination

2. Accumulation

3. Assimilation

Elimination occurs between four 4am till 12 noon. The body has already decided what goes where. Now it's the matter of extracting the waste products. For the most of us Americans we need to detoxify our intestines or in other words cleanse our intestines. The intestine tube is approximately twenty-four feet long in an adult body, so there is a lot of cleansing to do. The best way to go about this is by eating fruit and drinking fruit juice (not from concentrate) early in the morning until your bowel movements stabilize. You will experience more movements than normal. For about 2-4 weeks if you eat a lot of meat your bowels will stabilize to once in the morning and sometimes after lunch or dinner, depending on the fiber content of your meals. Just so you are sold on the process let me explain how it works.

The fruit juice and fruit is pre-digested therefore it does not require the digestion process, in other words it doesn't need to be broken down. Now the digestive and fruit enzymes are deployed to the stomach to assist in eliminating the waste from yesterday's meal(s). A tip, you should really eat four small meals a day not three big meals unless your work is physically demanding. The purpose of eating food is for energy not to satisfy taste buds. We will get more into that later on. So to recap the Elimination process starts everyday around 4am and ends around 12 noon to eliminate waste.

The second cycle is the Accumulation cycle which occurs between 12 noon and 8pm. This is the most important cycle because what we eat and how much determines how healthy we will be, including how much energy we'll have and how long our bodies will live. Therefore, be very conscious of what you eat and drink. There is usually more to what you eat than you may think. In the Accumulation cycle we are feeding our belly to strengthen it from disease and get energy to perform what we need and want to do. We will discuss this in another chapter. Your goal in this cycle should be to help your body stay healthy. Make no mistake about the importance of this cycle. This cycle will make or break you and none of us are exempt.

The third cycle is Assimilation. In this cycle the body goes to work dividing the good from the bad. This cycle starts about 8pm and lasts until about 4am. This is where your body stores carbohydrates, fat and protein for immediate and future use. During this cycle our body will separate the vitamins and minerals we need on a daily basis. This is our reactive cycle; it reacts to the accumulation cycle. This is why the accumulation cycle is so important. The body only has what we give it to work with. So now you know what your body is doing as you go through the day.

Please take a little time and answer these questions on the information in chapter one before you proceed to the next chapter. It's not what we read it's what we remember and do that counts.

1. How many cycles does the body have per day?

2. What is the order of the cycles and the time frames?

3. What happens in each cycle?

4. Which cycle is the most important?

5. List each cycle and our goal for each cycle.

6. How will we obtain our goal in each cycle?

This quiz concludes Chapter 1 of Body Smart 101.

CHAPTER 2
NUTRITION

Welcome to the nutrition chapter. In this chapter we will get you focused on and conscious of the nutrients you may be neglecting now. Here are your most important nutrients in the group.

- Water

- Fruit

- Vegetable

These nutrient rich sources I call the "Big Three", without any of them you're not eating a healthy diet. By the way a healthy diet is what you will eat from now on, not just for a short term. Short term diets don't work because you end up going back to your old habits, and usually end up gaining most of the weight back. Therefore, focus on changing your bad eating habits for good ones. Please take this information literally, you must change your eating habits to take advantage of this information.

Ok let's get going. First let's talk about water. Our bodies are about 65% water; if we do not maintain this percentage level we will become ill sooner or later. There is no substitute for water. Drink at least half your body weight in ounces per day. Of the big three water is the most important. Please let this book be your beginning, use the internet and your library to further study the information we are discussing.

Now let's talk about fruit, the second most important nutrient of the big three. This is the food that a lot of us Americans are missing. Fruit is the only food that is predigested. Fruit is what cleans the intestines. There is a secret you need to know about fruit, you should eat fruit on an empty stomach. This is because fruit is predigested and the fruit will rot if it runs into any other food already in the stomach. All the other foods have to be digested, therefore eat your fruit first so that it is not blocked in the stomach. The enzymes that are deployed to digest the fruit will go into the intestines to clean and extract any waste that has not been extracted already. So the next time you go to your grocery store buy some fruit. Make it a habit to eat a piece of fruit every two to three hours. As you go through the day remember that these habits will help you lose weight and get healthy. The only question is CAN YOU DO IT?

Now the third nutrient is the great vegetable. If you can make this nutrient the major player in all your meals, the potential for you being healthy and living longer are greatly increased. There is no debating that. The debate is CAN YOU DO IT? Know this about Body Smart, this book wasn't made to entertain you. This book is made to give you all the basics you need to win the battle of your health. We are challenged in this country like no other place in the world. So except the challenge and win the war. The great vegetable is one of the main nutrients you need. Here's a secret about vegetables you need to and probably already know, don't overcook them. They have living enzymes in them that will die if you overcook them. They are very different from meat, meat is dead when you eat it and vegetables are still alive. Therefore heat them carefully and at low temperatures.

This brings us to the end of chapter two. Next is the quick quiz and then on to chapter 3. As we did in chapter one please go through this quiz before going to chapter three.

1. What are the big three?

2. Which is the most important?

3. Which is the second most important?

4. The third important nutrient?

5. What is the range of percent of water in our bodies?

6. What is the secret to eating fruit?

7. What is the secret to eating vegetables?

CHAPTER 3
WHAT NOT TO EAT

What not to eat is almost as important as what to eat. Bad eating habits are what hurt us the most. If this book can only change one thing in your life, use it to change a bad habit into a good one. Here listed below are some of the things to avoid. Just to be clear the things that are discussed in this chapter will not harm you if eaten in moderation and sparingly, there are better choices available to us as Americans.

- White sugar

- Land animal meat

- White bread

Processed white sugar causes the blood sugar level to raise above normal levels at abnormal speeds and to drop in the same manor. Our bodies cannot calculate processed sugar. If you eat natural sugar your body calculates when it has had enough and it lets you know by giving you a full feeling. Many times we end up ingesting way too much processed sugar at one time. This action causes damage to our cells and our bodies have no choice but to store the excess sugar as fat. Abuse of processed sugar is one of the leading causes of obesity and diabetes.

In this chapter we need to discuss land animal meat. This is very important information. We as Americans eat way too much land animal meat. We should eat meat as a side dish, not the main dish. We do not need a lot of meat, let me tell you why. When you eat too much meat your body cannot digest it properly and some of the meat remains in your intesties, it's called fecal matter at that point. Eat a piece of fruit first then vegetables then your choice of meat, no more then four ounces.

The third thing not to eat is processed white bread. If the label says enriched or bleached the bread may be doing more harm than good. White bread is interesting in the way that the sugar in the white bread has explosive characteristics about it. Once the bread is in our bodies the sugar kind of explodes. So the amount of sugar on the label is not true, and we already discussed what happens with too much processed sugar. Choose whole wheat, rye or pumpernickel, they are much healthier choices. Your taste buds will change, and you will learn to enjoy these other bread choices.

Quiz

1. Name the first thing to avoid?

2. Name the second thing to avoid?

3. Name the third thing to avoid?

4. Why should you avoid sugar?

5. Why should you eat less land animal meat?

6. Why should you avoid white bread?

7. Should you research these things or take my word for it. Yes or no?

CHAPTER 4
WHAT TO EAT

This is a very important chapter. Many times we are either told to do the wrong thing or what not to do. In this chapter we will discuss what we should be eating. Here are your bullet points.

- Fruit

- Vegetables

- Fish

We have discussed fruit before, not only is fruit predigested and cleans the intestines but fruit also has nutritional value as well. Please do not let your study end here. Do a further research of all information in this book. I will give you the basics in this short book; it is up to you to get enough information to change your bad habits for good ones. Fruit has carbohydrates, protein and many other vitamins and minerals. If you are not eating fruit everyday you're not eating as healthy as you should. Your body deserves the best so give it the best.

The second super food here on our list is vegetables. I will tell you this if you can manage to make vegetables your main course of your four meals, your body will change internally. It will start to change immediately and continue to improve daily. My favorite reference is Dr. Decuypere's nutrient charts; there you will get great evidence of the benefits of vegetables and fruit. When we eat as we should our bodies will be full of nutrients and our blood will be rich in vitamins and minerals. Let me stop here and say if you are reading Body Smart, do as much research as you can need to convince yourself to change your eating habits for life. You are miles ahead of most Americans if you have gotten this far so don't go back.

Next is lean toward eating fish as a substitute for land animals meat. What I do is substitute a bad habit for a good one. Fish will increase your odds for a longer life span. It will also increase your odds of not enduring a heart attack. I've known doctors who have operated on people that have had heart attacks from consuming too much land animal meat. So let me tell you this, they would have done anything to avoid that so here is your chance to prevent it. Fish has omega 3's in them while land animals have omega 6's, big difference. Omega three's thin the blood and Omega six's make the blood thicker, O3's are from fish and O6's are from land animals. Fish will keep your blood thin while land meat makes your blood thick which is not good. Again don't let this be the end of your research, land meat vs. fish. The evidence is here, get it and change your life before it's too late. Also fish is not as fatty as land meat. Too much fat will kill the human body.

Quiz

1. What's the most important food?

2. Second most important?

3. Third most important?

4. What does fruit have in it?

5. What do vegetables have in them?

6. What do fish have in them?

7. Can you change your eating habits? Yes or no?

CHAPTER 5
EXERCISE

I will say that exercising is the most interesting of all. This chapter is also the most difficult to do. Let's define exercise. First exercise is any physical movement.

- What type of exercise?

- When is the best time?

- What is the benefit?

As far as type, the best exercise is the one you will do. Lots of people buy machines and get a membership to a gym but never get around to using either one. Therefore the best exercise is the one you enjoy doing. Most of us go home after work, eat, then sit down and watch TV. This is a great opportunity to change a bad habit into a good one. Look at exercise this way, the benefit is much greater than the cost. That's why it's so hard to do, like getting rich. Everyone wants to be rich but most of us aren't willing to do the work it takes. We can be physically rich or poor; it's a choice that you have to make. A wise man once said "the only thing that matters is what we can do and what we cannot do." After you finish reading Body Smart you will have the knowledge to become physically rich. There is no debate as to can you do it, the question is will you?

The best time to exercise is whenever you can. Cardio exercise is the hardest challenge you will face so come up with a game plan and do it. Make no mistake about it exercising builds physical wealth. That's why it's so hard to do. The rewards are great. Just like building a successful business, it's not going to be easy but you definitely can do it. You have to make exercising a priority in your life and make no excuses.

Why should I exercise is my third bullet point. Exercising makes your muscles stronger and last longer. Exercising builds up the internal body. Your blood pressure, heart rate, circulatory, respiratory and cardiovascular systems will become healthier.

Quiz

1. Define exercise.

2. What is the best exercise?

3. When is the best time to exercise?

4. How does exercising affect your health?

5. What is the benefit of exercise?

6. What qualifies as exercise?

7. Can you change and are you going to?

CHAPTER 6
IN THIS CHAPTER I WILL LIST ALL OF YOUR DAILY NUTRIENT REQUIREMENTS (D.R)

Before you read the requirements let me tell you this, your body needs protein and calcium everyday. If you fail to put either one of them in your body it will take the protein and calcium from your bones. Eventually your bones will become weak and brittle. Beans, Legumes, meat, fish and dairy products are excellent and available sources of protein and calcium.

1. Get some sweet potatoes, carrots, cantaloupe and dark green veggies.

2. Biotin D.V 300 micro grams/brewer's yeast, corn, barley, soybeans, walnuts, peanuts cauliflower, milk, egg yolk and fortified cereals.

3. Calcium D.V 1000 milligrams/ skim milk, nonfat yogurt and cheese, collard greens, mustard greens, kale, broccoli, canned salmon and sardines with bones, corn tortillas processed with lime calcium, fortified orange juice.

4. Folic acid D.V 400 micrograms/ fortified cereal, pinto beans navy beans, asparagus, spinach, broccoli and Brussels sprouts.

5. Iron D.V 18 milligrams/ beef, cream of wheat cereal, baked potatoes, soybeans and pumpkin seeds.

6. Magnesium D.V 400 milligrams/ brown rice, avocado's, spinach, haddock, oatmeal, baked potatoes, navy beans, lima beans, broccoli, yogurt and bananas.

7. Niacin D.V 20 milligrams/ chicken breast, tuna, fortified breads and cereals.

8. Pantothenic Acid D.V 10 milligrams/ whole grain, mushrooms, salmon and peanuts.

9. Phosphorus D.V 100 milligrams/ halibut, nonfat yogurt, salmon, skim milk, chicken breast, oatmeal, extra lean ground beef, broccoli and lima beans.

10. Potassium D.V 3500 milligrams/ dried apricots, baked potatoes, dried prunes, cantaloupe, bananas and spinach.

11. Riboflavin D.V 1.7 milligrams/ poultry fish, fortified grains and cereals, broccoli, turnip greens, asparagus, spinach, yogurt, milk and cheese.

12. Selenium D.V 70 micrograms/ lobster, Brazil nuts, clams, crab, cooked oysters and whole grains.

13. Sodium D.V 2400 milligrams/ cottage cheese, canned soups, canned veggies, shellfish, canned tuna, baked goods and salad dressing.

14. Sulfur D.V non fish and poultry

15. Thiamin D.V 1.5 milligrams/ rice, bran, fresh peas', beans, whole grain, oranges, oatmeal and some cereals.

16. Trace minerals boron D.V none parsley, apples, cherries, grapes, leafy veggies, nuts and beans

17. Chromium D.V 120 micrograms/ brewer's yeast, broccoli, grape juice (not from concentrate)

18. Cobalt D.V none fish

19. Copper D.V 2 milligrams/ shellfish, cooked oysters, nuts, seeds, coco powder, beans, whole grains and mushrooms.

20. Fluorine D.V 1.5 milligrams water

21. Iodine D.V 150 micrograms iodized salt, lobster, shrimp, cooked oyster, marine fish, seaweed breads and milk

22. Magnesium D.V 2 milligrams/ canned pineapple juice, wheat, bran, whole grain, seeds, nuts, coco, shellfish and tea

23. Molybdenum D.V 75 micrograms/ beans, whole grain, cereal, milk and milk products. Dark green leafy veggies.

24. Vitamin A D.V 5000 international units/ carrot juice(not from concentrate), pumpkin, sweet potatoes, carrots, spinach, butternut squash, tuna, dandelion greens, cantaloupe, mangos, turnip greens and beet greens

25. Vitamin B6 D.V 2 milligrams/ bananas, avocados, eggs, brown rice, soy beans, oats, whole wheat, peanuts and walnuts

26. Vitamin B12 D.V 6 micrograms/ clams, cooked oysters, king crab, herring, salmon and tuna

27. Vitamin C D.V 60 milligrams/ pineapple, broccoli, peppers, cantaloupe, strawberries, kiwi and pink grapefruit

28. Vitamin D D.V 400 international units/ herring, salmon, sardines, fortified milk, eggs and fortified cereals

29. Vitamin E D.V 30 int. units/ veggies, nuts, oil, soybean, corn, whole grains, wheat germ and spinach

30. Vitamin K D.V 80 micrograms/ cauliflower, broccoli, green leafy veggies, spinach and kale

31. Zinc D.V 15 milligrams/ cooked oysters, eggs, whole grain, nuts and yogurt

That's it folks, it may seem like a lot but it's not. If you noticed some of the foods have several of the vitamins and minerals that you need. I think we covered enough in this chapter so stop and review for about half an hour. For most of you this is the first time you've seen all the daily values at one time.

Here is a technique for you that's easy and effective! Take a multi-vitamin until you can figure out a meal menu that has all the daily nutrients in them, in Body Smart 102 I will have menu's with one third of the daily values for a three meal a day plan.

What I do when I take college courses is I give myself a final project. I go above and beyond the requirements of the course. This has been a successful habit for me and will be for you also. So what I'm suggesting is that as a final project you create a daily menu for yourself based on chapter 6. This is something we all should do for every month all year round. Remember this book is not for your entertainment, its purpose is to help change your daily habits. So please just do it and don't make excuses, it's up to you don't fail yourself. They say we remember the first and last things we hear so I saved the best for last. Have you ever heard of DR. Hippocrates of Kos (CA 460 BC—CA 370 BC) Greece. He is referred to as the father of western medicine. Please research him and the Hippocratic Oath. My favorite statement "let food be your medicine and your medicine be your food.

Now add exercise to that and you will be the champion of your own and your families' health.

Good Health to you all!

Printed in the United States
By Bookmasters